PUPPY TRAINING

Top 50 Proven Tips and Tricks to Raise A Dream Dog

Jane Wolfe

Copyright © 2017 by Jane Wolfe

All rights reserved. No part of this publication may be reproduced, distributed or transmitted in any form or by any means, without prior written permission from the author.

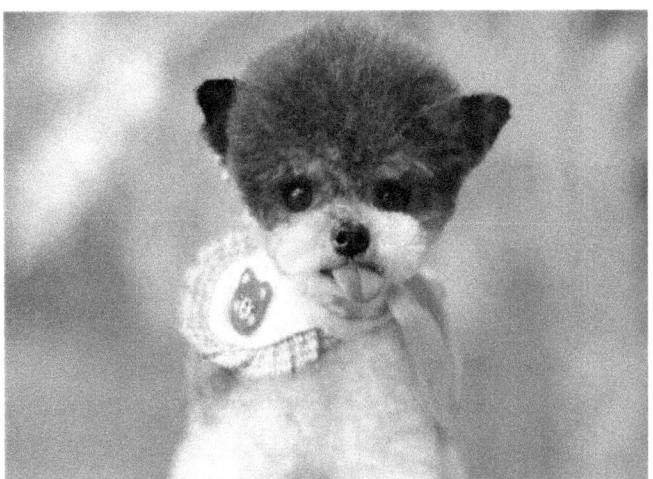

Table of Contents

Introduction 1

Chapter 1: Puppy Crate Training Basics 3

Chapter 2: Puppy Toilet Training Essentials 8

Chapter 3: Puppy Socialization Fundamentals 14

Chapter 4: Resolving Your Puppy's Separation Anxiety Issues 18

Chapter 5: Leading Your Future Dream Dog 22

Chapter 6: Managing Canine Behavioral Problems 26

Chapter 7: Canine Health and Safety Necessities 35

Chapter 8: Your Obedience Training Guide 46

Chapter 9: Surviving Your Puppy's First Day at Home .. 50

Conclusion 60

Introduction

I want to thank you and congratulate you for downloading the book, "Puppy Training: Top 50 Proven Tips and Tricks to Raise A Dream Dog".

This book contains proven steps and strategies on how to effectively guide and groom your puppy into the dream dog you have always wanted.

This book will prepare you for one of the biggest surprises of your life - molding your puppy into your future dream dog is not just about tossing him treats and making him sit without a peep while you watch television. Within the pages of this book, you will discover the difficulties of successfully rearing a puppy into a well-adjusted adult dog-hood.

This book contains various tips and tricks to help your puppy get cozy in his crate, eliminate without a hitch, bond easily with people and other dogs, feel secured when separated from you, and acknowledge you as is leader. You will also learn from this book how to manage disobedience and other misbehavior problems as well as how to ensure your puppy's safety and health. You even get to learn how to make your puppy's first day at home as painless and as enjoyable as possible.

Happy puppy rearing!

Chapter 1

Puppy Crate Training Basics

One way of ensuring that your pup grows up into a well-behaved dog is crate training him properly. Follow these 5 tips and tricks on crate training your soon-to-be dream dog.

1. Avoid treating the crate as your puppy's magic box.

- Use the crate correctly to meet your puppy's needs. Although the crate will certainly be a big help to you in housetraining your puppy, it is not a magical solution to all your puppy problems. Your puppy may tend to feel frustrated and trapped inside his crate, if you fail to use it the proper way.

  Avoid crating your dog the whole day you are working out of the house, then putting him inside the crate again the entire night. You are just forcing your dog to spend too much of his time in such a small space. Keep your puppy's physical as well as emotional needs in mind, especially if he is still below six months old. He should not be confined in his crate for periods that are longer than three to four hours, since he still has not developed the ability to control his bladder and bowels for a long time.

- Make sure the crate is made with the right materials. You have the option to use a metal crate that is of the collapsible type, or a plastic crate normally used as a flight kennel. You can get a puppy crate from pet supply stores, and there are a wide range of sizes to choose from that will fit your dog's needs.

  Make sure your puppy's crate is big enough to accommodate him while standing up and when turning around inside it. It would be wise to get a crate that will accommodate your puppy during his growing up period until his adulthood. If the crate is still too big for your puppy, see to it that any excess space is blocked off to keep him from urinating or defecating on one side, and then retreating to the other side.

2. Help your puppy see how wonderful his crate is.

- Gradually coax your dog into his crate. Make the crate look inviting by placing small food treats close to it at first. Once your puppy goes near the crate as he grabs the treats, start dropping the treats inside the crate door until you are dropping treats further inside the crate.

  Don't worry if your dog does not want to enter the crate at first. You should avoid forcing your dog to enter his crate. Just go continue placing his treats inside the crate; eventually, you will find him nonchalantly entering the crate all the way in so that he can have the food.

If your puppy does not seem to care for food treats one way or another, his favorite toy may work to reel him in. Remember that encouraging your dog to get inside his crate can take a few minutes to several days. It would take a little practice so you need to be patient during this stage.

- Take advantage of the command-and-treat technique. Use a regular command, followed by a treat, to have your puppy enter his crate. You may find it easier to place the crate in the bedroom hallway or inside your room at first. Your puppy will need to frequently urinate or defecate during the night, and having him nearby will ensure that you can hear him whining to be let out of his crate.

3. Let your dog enjoy his meal inside the crate.

As soon as your puppy can comfortably stand inside his crate as he eats his meal, you may let him go on eating as you close the door. Start by opening the door the moment he is done with his meal. You can then move on to successively leaving the crate door closed several minutes longer, until your puppy can stay inside the crate for ten minutes or longer after he is done eating his meal.

In case he whines and begs to get out of the crate, it only means that you are making him stay longer too quickly. The next time you try to train your dog to use his crate, let him stay inside for a shorter time; if he still whines, hold your ground this time and don't let him out of the crate unless he stops whining. This will help him see that whining will not be his ticket out of the crate.

4. Fill your dog's crate with safe toys for him to play with when you are out.

Once your puppy can comfortably spend about half an hour inside his crate without anxiety or fear, you can start crating him for short periods of time, like when you need to get out of the house. Use your regular command to let him inside the crate, then reward him with a treat. Or try leaving some of his favorite toys in the crate before going out. Make sure to change the times of the day when you let your dog inside his crate, so he doesn't assume it is a routine. Keep in mind that you can crate your dog about five to twenty minutes before you leave the house.

5. Don't encourage any whining in the crate.

You may encounter a little difficulty knowing whether your crated puppy cries at night because he wants to get out of the crate or because he needs to go outside to urinate or defecate. This is a good thing, because it means that you have not rewarded your puppy in the past for whining by letting him out of his crate. The best you can do is to try letting his whining pass without giving attention to it. Scolding, shouting, or pounding will only make your puppy whine louder and more intensely; your puppy will stop whining soon if you ignore him.

Chapter 2

Puppy Toilet Training Essentials

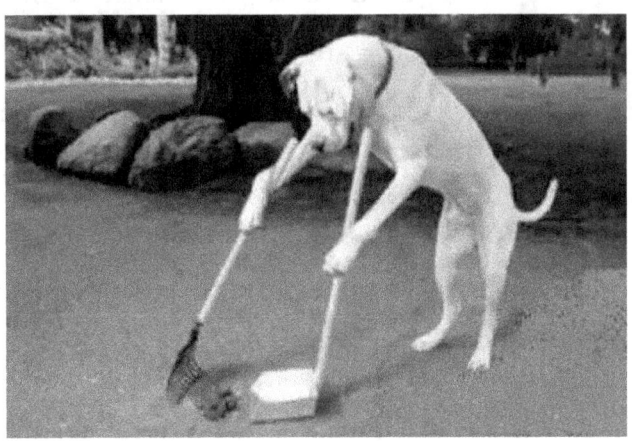

No fuss, no mess – you wish. But these 5 easy-to-follow puppy toilet training tips and tricks will help nudge your puppy in the right potty direction.

1. Take steps to make the toilet training ride as smooth as possible.

- Keep in mind that your puppy won't be able to hold his urge to go for long periods of time. The same goes even for adult dogs; they still could use the help of a dog walker in the middle of the day. Your puppy would need to urinate and defecate on regularly, which is why you need to ensure that he gets to go out to get toilet trained at least every four hours.

- Get rid of any opportunity for toilet training accidents to happen. Make sure to have your puppy near you during his first fourteen days. This way, once he begins urinating or defecating indoors, you are there to correct him right away. If you fail to do this, your puppy might relieve himself in other parts of the house.

  Even if you scold him to no end afterwards, if you did not catch your puppy in the act, it would be useless since he cannot remember what he did or understand to make the connection of your anger to what he might have done. Make sure to keep any unused rooms closed off. To keep your puppy beside you, keep him leashed. Either hold the leash or attach it to furniture. It also helps to crate your puppy whenever you are out of the house.

- Keep your eyes peeled for circling, restlessness, and other signs of your puppy's discomfort. Once you do spot his discomfort, immediately take him outside to the nearby potty place you have established. In case your puppy urinates or defecates in the wrong spot, realize that it is not because of spitefulness.

  It only means that he really had to. If you cannot immediately take your puppy outside, you will have to deal with a big problem later – because your puppy has realized that relieving himself indoors once he feels the urge to go feels so good, he is more likely to keep on doing so.

- Confine your puppy if you cannot watch him. You may put your puppy in a crate or in a designated spot in your kitchen. Never leave any food lying around, but make sure to leave water, especially if he only is confined inside the crated or confined in the designated kitchen spot for no more than two hours. Treat the crate or kitchen spot as your puppy's domain until he is properly toilet trained.

2. Help your puppy along in his potty routine.

- Have your puppy eat on schedule. Fifteen minutes after feeding your puppy at regular times every day, take him outside to do his thing. You can usually feed your young pup thrice a day, while you can feed older puppies (as well as adult dogs) two times a day. See to it that you are keeping your dog's diet consistent, as switching up his foods will make it more difficult for you to training him.

- Have your puppy follow a potty routine. Establish a regular routine for your puppy. You can let your puppy out of his crate to go outside to eliminate the moment he wakes up, within one hour after he has his meal, once you arrive from work, after a physical activity, and right before his bedtime. If your puppy is quite young, you may have to let him put every two hours. Keep in mind that housebreaking your puppy will be quicker and more effective if you see to it that he is taken out in the middle of the day.

3. Know that punishment is not the answer to your puppy's toilet troubles.

- Be gentle with your dog. Never punish your puppy for answering his need to go. Don't, under any circumstances, smack him or shove his nose into the mess he made. You will only be teaching him to fear hands this way. A dog forgets the things he does after doing them, so he cannot relate any of his past actions to a punishment you might be giving him at that moment. He will learn, however, to associate anger and pain with you, the person who is inflicting pain as a form of punishment.

- Think big voice over physical force. When you catch your puppy misbehaving, try interrupting him by letting out a loud "No!" As soon as he gets startled into stopping whatever he is doing, bring him to his spotty spot. Make sure to avoid muttering or repeating your command – using a deep and loud voice would be more effective in getting your message across.

- Don't skimp on the praise. Whenever your puppy goes potty, make sure to reward him with praise. To reinforce the good behavior, let him have a kibble or other treat. In case he still does not go after fifteen or so minutes have gone, bring him inside the house for about five minutes before bringing him outside again.

4. Don't associate walking your dog outside with his potty schedule.

Avoid ending your walks outside whenever your puppy decides to urinate or defecate. This will only give him the idea that any outdoor fun he engages in comes to a halt when he need to go potty. This is also the reason there are dogs that hold their urge to eliminate until they get home. As soon as your puppy eliminates, reward him with praise, a treat, and some more walking.

5. Keep it clean for your puppy's sake.

Never leave a mess after your puppy goes potty, whether inside the house or out in his potty spot. To keep him from thinking that eliminating is a form of interactive play, make sure he does not see you clean up after him. Get rid of any urine smells with pet odor neutralizer made with an enzyme base.

Chapter 3

Puppy Socialization Fundamentals

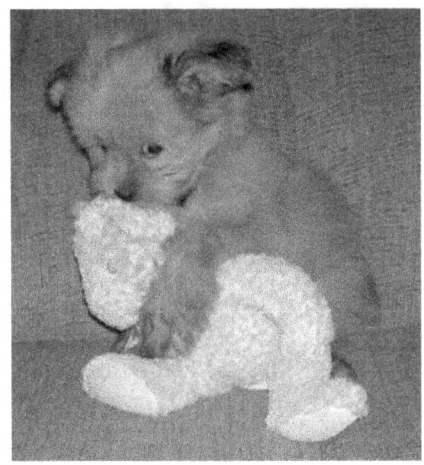

Allow your puppy to get used to various situations and prepare him for challenges in the future by teaching him fundamental socialization skills. Here are 5 tips and tricks to guide you:

1. Keep things light.

- Use the leash to make the social connection. Introduce your puppy to one person or dog/other animal at a time, with the help of his leash for control. Make sure to exercise him to calm him down before any meeting; it also helps to have handy treats to encourage as well as reward your puppy for behaving well. Using a leash will also help you immediately correct him as needed. To make introductions go even more smoothly, act confident around your puppy, and see to it that the visitor is relaxed.

- Make sure to give attention to the resident dog by petting him. This will also assure him that everything will be all right with his meeting with your puppy. If things do not go as you hoped they would, it might be better to put off the meeting and introduce them again some other time.

2. Practice damage control, especially when introducing your pup to other dogs.

- Make sure your puppy and the dog you are introducing him to are within each other's sight. If introducing your puppy to three or more dogs, let him meet one dog at a time. If you find the animals receiving each other well, don't hesitate to pet, praise, and give a treat to each dog – this shows them that being with each other will allow good things to happen.

- Keep an eye on stiffening up, staring, back-fur rising, and other warning signs. Never punish one dog reacting to the other in an aggressive way. It would be better for you to bring him to somewhere he could be alone; allow him to settle down and then ignore him. Do the same with each dog if they both start acting aggressively. You may then introduce them again some other time.

3. Remember that timing is everything.

- Timing is important when it comes to correcting any dog behavior that is unacceptable. Avoid waiting for one dog to lunge at the other. As soon as you sense any hint of aggression, immediately correct him by firmly saying "No" as you yank the leash for correction, not punishment. This will bring the aggressor's attention to you and get the message across that you are the leader of the pack. You have no reason to feel alarmed if your puppy does not warm up to other dogs right away; otherwise, especially if this goes on more than one to two weeks, a consultation with a dog specialist may be in order.

- It usually takes days or weeks for dogs to acclimatize, so give your puppy about ten to fifteen minutes of daily quality time with you. Play with your dog, give him a massage, brush his coat, and practice different training skills with him. As soon as your puppy reacts well to other dogs, you may then remove their leashes. You will still need to watch over them though, and keep a whistle or spray bottle around to distract them when they start showing aggression. It also helps to have treats on hand for rewarding good behavior.

4. Allow your puppy to ease into the socialization training process.

Your puppy may feel stressed and overwhelmed with surrounding changes, which is why getting him introduced to too many people is not such a good idea. Delay any socialization until your puppy gets settled in his surroundings than risk having him constantly nip or cower whenever he meets other people.

5. Make room for difficulties along the way.

You can expect your puppy to act like one – he will likely growl, jump on people, and engage in other behaviors that need correction. It also helps to ask other people to refrain from playing biting, tug of war, wrestling, or any aggressive game with your dog.

Chapter 4

Resolving Your Puppy's Separation Anxiety Issues

Your puppy always seems anxious when you are out of the house – understandably, he just wants to be with you all the time. But there are 5 simple tips and tricks to deal around this problem:

1. Let your dog cozy up in his crate first.

Provide your puppy a haven when you are away by teaching him to stay in his crate. Make it cozy to live in by placing a comfortable bedding inside, as well as some safe dog toys. You can also feed your puppy while he is inside his crate, as this lets him see that good things happen inside his crate. When he does stay in the crate, reward him with praise and treats.

You can also let your puppy get cozy in a spot in the hallway or kitchen. Just make sure it is confined within baby gates. You may need to place two gates on top of one another if your puppy tends to jump.

2. Give some leeway for your dog to express his anxiety.

- You can place a chew toy (made of rubber) inside your puppy's crate to give him something to chew his separation anxiety away with. Try smearing some peanut butter inside the toy – this will encourage your puppy to lick for hours. Dry kibble is another fun anxiety outlet for your puppy to play with.

- When it is time for you to leave, say "Good dog!" in a quiet tone. Then give you puppy a small treat before leaving immediately. You don't have to say goodbye to your puppy – just walk away. When you come back, praise him by saying "Good dog!" again in a quiet tone before taking him out.

- See to it that your puppy is not left alone for long periods, especially if you do not want any accidents to happen when you are out. It would be a good idea to hire someone to walk your puppy in the middle of the day.

3. Step back for a while.

- Avoid spending the entire day with your puppy the first time you bring him home. Let him into his crate with his bed, water, and chew toys waiting for him. Ask him to lie down, then praise him and give him a treat as you call him by his name. Make sure he realizes that you are pleased with what he just did by stepping away; if he starts getting restless, immediately bring him outside for a walk or to play.

- When placing your puppy back in his crate, immediately step away and stay in another room. Come back only after some time has passed. You can then leave the house and return immediately, eventually making your trip longer with each practice. This will teach your puppy to feel less anxious whenever you leave, because he knows you would return after a while.

4. Teach your dog to trust you.

Place a treat inside your puppy's crate to coax him into entering it. Once he is inside, talk to him and let him feel comfortable inside. This will help your puppy learn to trust you as well as know that you are the one who decides what to do.

5. Count on exercise to calm your puppy down.

Make sure your puppy gets plenty of exercise before leaving the house. About twenty minutes before going out, do what you usually do in a calm manner, and then leave without making a fuss as you say goodbye to your dog.

Chapter 5

Leading Your Future Dream Dog

Your puppy needs a leader to guide him into becoming a dream dog, not a human to dominate. Get the stress, confusion, and aggression out of the way by teaching your dog to see you as the one in charge – with these 5 tips and tricks.

1. Give up the freebies.

- Your puppy must learn from now on that in to get in your good graces and receive the enjoyable treats, delicious meals, praises, petting, and walks, he should be on his best behavior. Use the good things in your dog's life as rewards for good behavior, and you will have an easier time leading him.

- Prior to setting down your puppy's food bowl, command your puppy to "Sit," and do so only once. He will only be able to eat his food – after you praise him with an enthusiastic "Good boy!" – when he calmly sits. Make sure that he sits properly, not bouncing up and down in one spot. Make him see that there is no way he could eat if he does not sit. If your puppy still does not sit, take his food bowl away, and then try the process later. If you and your puppy eat at the same time, make sure he sees you eat your meal first before placing his own food down. He needs to realize that you get to eat first because you are the leader.

2. Always lead, all the way.

- You should keep your puppy from bolting ahead of you when walking, and he should not be dragging you out the door, either. Make sure to keep him on a leash and ask him to sit; then, walk out the door first. Not until he sits and stays, do not give him the chance to go out. If he tries to barrel through the door as you are opening it, immediately shut it every time his nose is about to reach the opening. Do these five to six times or until he gets the whole idea.

- Make sure you are staying on a level that is higher than your puppy. Avoid sitting down when you pet him, and refrain from playing with him on the floor. Pet him and give him praise from any high level above his head. Until your dog learns to acknowledge you as his leader, don't allow him on any furniture, especially on your bed.

- When making eye-to-eye contact with your dog, act like the leader you are and hold your stare long enough to make him turn his eyes away.

3. Know when to pay attention and when to ignore.

Jumping is a form of dominating behavior, which is why you should discourage your puppy from doing it. You can command him to stop with a form "No" or "Off", or ignore him. You can also try greeting your dog or petting him only when he stops jumping and begins to sit still.

4. Let everyone in on the leading action.

Your puppy should not be encouraged to play favorites among members of the household. Anyone who is ignored or intimidated by the puppy should be the one given the task to feed the puppy as well as give him treats. It is also important that every member of the household does this task as the puppy gets housetrained.

5. Use your puppy's crate to send the message that you are his leader.

Teach your puppy to willingly get inside his crate; when you command him to do so, never take "no" for a reply.

Turn the crate into a welcoming spot by rewarding him with treats for entering it. It also helps to feed him while he is inside the crate. Keeping your dog inside the crate for about an hour before his training session also ensures that he directs his undivided attention on you. This technique also teaches your dog that you are the leader, and that you are the one who decides when he enters and gets out of the crate. Ignore your dog if he starts barking while in the crate. Release him only once he is relaxed and quiet.

Chapter 6

Managing Canine Behavioral Problems

Your puppy has a natural tendency to engage in "bad' behavior. But this does not mean you should let him be and then wreck his chances of growing up into your dream dog – not if you follow these 10 behavioral problem management tips and tricks.

1. Wait it out.

You will find that it might take a while before you are able to train your puppy, as well as trust him enough to let him move about freely inside the house. You can expect that to happen after a few weeks. Before it does happen, you can safely confine your puppy in his crate (or a bay-gated area in the kitchen), especially when you can't watch over him. Make sure to leave some of his favorite toys in the crate, and keep all trash cans out of sight.

2. Allow your puppy to be active.

His excess energy, that is. You might think there is something wrong about your puppy being so active. Dogs need to engage in exercise as well as to be paid attention to. If you are unable to give both to your puppy, he has no choice but to spend his extra energy somewhere else. And keep in mind that dogs are not like humans, who may do certain things to spite someone else - your puppy acts hyperactive because it is his way of coping with all that energy.

3. Get at the root of the behavior problem.

Your dog's undesirable behavior can frequently be caused by the frustration he feels for being left alone, especially since dogs by nature, are social animals. Try having him watched over by a dog walker (midday) or placing him in a doggie day care facility if you need to leave him on his own for long periods. Misbehavior in dogs can also stem from stress between family members or the arrival of a new member, while some behavior problems in dogs may be a call for modifications in their diet.

4. Make sure your puppy is caught in the misbehaving act.

Your puppy cannot remember any recent activity he has done, which is why you should be there to catch and correct him when he misbehaves.

5. Manage your puppy's chewing issues.

- Your puppy's tendency to chew is a means for him to explore his surroundings (adult dogs chew for stress relief). To correct this behavior, make sure that any chewable object is out of your puppy's reach – hide the throw rugs, get power cords out of the way, and cover furniture legs with bitter apple spray. It also helps to allow your puppy easy access to his favorite chew toys, although you should limit the number to keep him from thinking he could have everything. When your puppy plays with the right chew toy, then you can give him a reward. You should also find the time to exercise your puppy as well as help him learn obedience commands so he has outlets for his energy.

- Command your puppy to drop or leave the off-limits object right away the moment you see him chewing it. Before you do this, you need to teach him the same command using positive reinforcement. As soon as your puppy does drop or leave the object, make sure to heap on the praises, and reward him with a suitable chewing substitute.

- Let your puppy learn the art of releasing objects from his mouth. Attach your puppy's leash and training collar before giving him one of his favorite toys. Next, hold his leash with your left hand while keeping a slack hold on his training collar, and issue the "Drop it" command. Remove the object from his mouth right away and praise him by saying "Good dog!"

- If you catch your puppy baring teeth or locking eyes, give his training collar a single yank, then let go. Act enthusiastic as you give him praises when he drops the object. But if your dog acts aggressive, keep yourself from smacking him (you may seek a professional's help instead), or he may perceive this to be threatening and bite you in instinctive response.

6. Put a lid on your dog's barking troubles.

- Some dog breeds are bred to bark. If your puppy happens to be that breed, you need to know his barking triggers. His trigger could be kids going through the door after school, the mail carrier stopping by, a neighbor mowing his yard, or a couple of joggers doing their daily routine – make sure to reduce his opportunities to encounter any of these trigger events.

- It would be a wise thing to immediately bring your puppy indoors before the above-mentioned trigger events take place. Shielding him this way makes it less likely for him to bark in response. Avoid giving your puppy the perception that his barking caused the triggers to leave.

- If there is no way for you to prevent the trigger events from taking place, you have to take steps to divert his attention towards you and away from the triggers. This can be easily accomplished by giving your puppy small treats as well as praising him. You might also try giving him a quick yank by the leash before he has the chance to focus on the barking target. Stop your puppy before he even begins to bark; immediately say "Quiet!" As soon as he looks at you, give him praises and treats. Follow through on this strategy to ensure teaching him that not barking is better than barking.

7. Break your puppy's jumping habit.

- Ask people to refrain from exciting your puppy too much that he starts jumping. If your puppy does jump, the best way to stop the behavior is to simply ignore him and walk away. When he calmly sits on command, provide him treats and your undivided attention.

- Avoid leaving your puppy by himself the entire day or night. This will often result in your puppy developing into a nervous, jumpy dog. Dogs labeled as problematic have usually been kept in basements or outdoors (the latter makes him likely to jump over the fence for escape).

- Dogs, being naturally inclined to go with fellow dogs, can get bored, lonely, and into mischief if left alone. If going out of the house, make sure to leave your puppy in a part of your home where the family usually hangs out. Confine him first in the crate or in a spot cornered by baby gates; once he has been properly house-trained, you can then let him freely move about.

- Your puppy would rather have you as playmate over a big yard to jump around in. Take time to really be with your dream dog – his needs for socialization and mental stimulation can also benefit from your active companionship.

8. Keep your puppy off the furniture.

- Hogging the furniture is a behavior problem that can be resolved with consistency in training. Let your puppy learn to get off the furniture by attaching to his collar a long leash whenever you are home; make sure to leave the leash on only during those times you are together in one room. The moment you puppy gets on the furniture, quickly correct him with the leash. It is important to prevent your dog from hopping onto furniture since the elevation gives him a sense of leadership and nudges him into showing aggression. Steer your puppy towards his comfy crate and bedding instead.

- To make it possible to keep your puppy from hopping onto furniture when you are away, strategically place balloons or large bubble wrap on them. The popping sounds these items make, which dogs do not like to hear – will effectively keep him away.

- Your puppy has a better chance of not getting into trouble if you keep him on his leash around the house. However, for his safety, don't forget to remove the leash when you leave him unattended for even a minute.

9. Control your dog's clinging tendencies.

- Your puppy can initially act shy or needy around you. If the transition period has passed and he still clings to you or another family member, use vocal praise and tasty treats to coax him into going near other family members. You can let others do the petting, feeding, and walking so that your puppy gradually feels safe and happy around them.

- Never stay silent around your clingy, shy puppy. Be generous with vocal praise, support, and encouragement.

- You can try setting up situations designed to make your dog win if he behaves properly. Refuse to pet him and focus your attention away from him if he acts all shy and clingy, then shower him with plenty of praise, hugs and treats when he switches to another appropriate behavior.

10. Nip your puppy's biting problems in the bud.

- Contrary to what some would say, biting and nipping are not puppy behaviors. If you do not correct this unacceptable behavior right from the start, you will be facing future biting and nipping incidents that will only get worse with time. Nipping and biting are usually used by dogs to test their owner's limits, and to find out who truly is the leader. Absence of socialization skills, feelings of dominance, fear, unbalanced diet, serious health problems, and role confusion (within the pack) also play a role in a dog' biting tendencies. Seek the help of your vet or another dog professional so that this behavior is immediately corrected.

- Make sure to set limits on your dog – you are his leader. Keep yourself from asking your puppy to follow a command to sit or stay, then act delighted with the fact that he looks so cute when he jumps on the couch. Always give your puppy a reward when he obeys and correct him without fail when he refuses to.

- Nipping during playtime is still unacceptable behavior. If your puppy tries this, firmly say "No' and stop the game right away. You can pull at his leash for correction as well to send the message that what he is doing is not right. Say "Good dog" the moment he stops nipping and calms down. Make sure to call him by his name when giving him praise, but never use it when correcting him. It also helps to provide your puppy a chew toy to nip instead of your hand.

Chapter 7

Canine Health and Safety Necessities

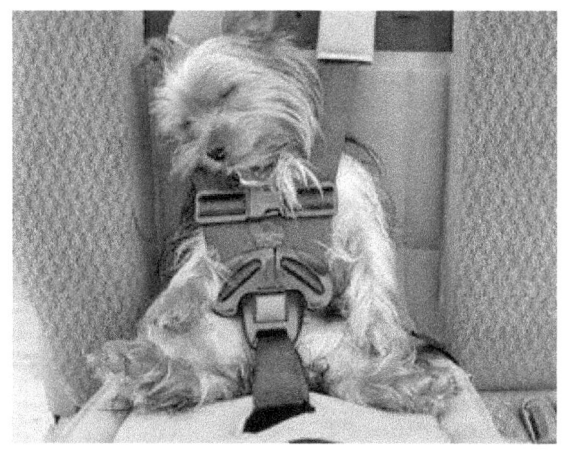

Keeping your puppy healthy and safe means ensuring that he grows and lives up to being the dream dog you have always wanted. Follow these 5 tips and tricks on ensuring your pup's health and safety so you can rest easy.

1. See the vet right away.

The best time to go see the veterinarian is sooner than later. Make sure to bring your puppy's medical records with you when you do see the vet. Ask to have your dog undergo thorough physical examinations to check for heartworm and other health conditions. And see your vet right away when your housetrained puppy continues having accidents.

2. Have your puppy's medical checklist on hand.

- Make sure your dog is complete with all the necessary shots.
- Follow your vet's recommendations for flea prevention and tick control.
- Ask your vet about heartworm prevention.
- Have the vet check your puppy for parasites if he seems preoccupied with his anal area.
- Check for red eyes, a sign of allergies or conjunctivitis.
- Brush your dog's teeth no less than four times per week.
- Examine your dog's ears and clean them once per week.
- Pay attention to your puppy's toes on a regular basis for any debris.

3. Take care of your pup at home.

- Diarrhea: Your pup could use some rice liquid after suffering from diarrhea. Cook rice with more water than usual, turning off the heat before the rice grains absorb all the liquid. Pour the starchy liquid into a small bowl and give to your puppy.

- Fleas and ticks: Check with your vet for recommendation on effective flea and tick control. There are topical flea or tick control liquid products that you can apply every three months. You may also give monthly oral tablets and try to keep fleas and ticks at bay (mechanisms include killing the adult parasites, preventing the eggs from hatching, or acting as heartworm preventative at the same time).

- Ear problems: To make sure your puppy's ears are thoroughly cleaned and healthy, you need to regularly remove any wax, dirt, or excess moisture. Combine 1 part of white vinegar with 1 part of lukewarm water, then pour into the dog's ear while lightly massaging the ear's base so that the solution is evenly distributed. Wipe-clean the outer ear with a cotton ball. After letting your puppy shake out any excess liquid, use a dry cotton ball to clean the ear. Repeat the process as needed. For problems like having an object lodged inside the ear, foul odor/discharge, swelling, redness, scratching, excessive tenderness, debris, or head-shaking, you should immediately see the vet for proper treatment.

- Heartworm: The treatment of heartworm disease is so difficult on dogs, which is why it is important to prevent it by any means possible. Heartworms refer to lethal mosquito-transmitted parasites that can cause multiple organ (liver, kidney, and lung) failure and death. Protect your puppy from heartworm disease by simply getting monthly pills from the vet, seeing to it that your puppy does not miss a single dose of preventative, and having him undergo a blood test to check for possible infection.

4. Learn effective dog-proofing and safety techniques.

- Doggie doors: Make sure the doggie doors are blocked whenever you leave the house or are unable to watch your puppy.

- Screen doors: Block all screen doors, which your puppy can tear through or kick open without any difficulty.

- Fences: Fences can have bent edges at the bottom, loose boards, or gaps that can easily hurt your puppy, so repair them right away. Place any woodpiles in an area far from the fences. And never leave your dog unattended when let out in the yard – he could break through the fence pickets, or dig under, jump over, or climb the fences and escape.

- Electric fences (invisible): Although electric fences are convenient for you and your family, they emit shocks that can be a health hazard to your dog. During a power failure, he could go over the electric fences and run off to get injured. Some dogs also learn to ignore the shocks so that they could go after other animals or people who are passing by.

- Open stairs or railings: You can install puppy gates or baby gates to block any open stairs or railings in the house.

- Latches on gates: See to it that your dog is unable to open any of the gate latches.

- Cold weather: Never let your dog stay out of the house when the weather is cold. He could get frostbite, damage his paw pads by stepping on rock salt, and get ill from the toxic effects of ice melt licked off from his paws. When walking your dog, make sure to get rid of any ice balls lodged between his toes afterwards, before wiping both his feet using damp towels.

- Hot weather: It is important to never leave your puppy alone in the car, and more so when the weather is hot. The temperature inside your car can easily go up, even when you open the windows, and cause death of an unattended dog.

- Weed killer: After applying weed killer to your yard, make sure to keep your puppy from stepping on the grass. He could lick his paws later and get sick.

- Heatstroke: Leaving your puppy out for a long time on hot days leaves him susceptible to heatstroke. Make sure your dog has access to plenty of water and a shady shelter whenever he is let out of the house.

- Transport: When transporting your dog, avoid placing him at the back, especially if you are driving a pickup truck. Doing so can cause your dog to fall out of the truck and die. If you are going to transport him in a car, you still should not be placing him in the back – he could stick his head out the window and get his eyes or head injured.

- Cleaning products: You can also install childproof latches on low cabinets, or hide all your cleaning products behind latched doors or in high cabinets

- Bones: Bones may splinter, get lodged in your puppy's throat or stomach, and cause deadly punctures. A good alternative to letting your puppy chew on bones is to let him play with dog rubber bones.

- Toilet: Keep your dog from drinking from the toilet, which may have toxic chemical traces from the tank/bowl freshener.

- Chains and ropes: Never use chains and ropes to secure your puppy to one place. These can easily injure your puppy and even prevent him from protecting himself when stray animals get near him. Keep in mind that chaining a dog can cause them to feel frustrated, leading to the development of behavioral problems like aggression.

- Chocolate: Chocolate is poison for your puppy – do not give him any, not even a lick.

- Aspirin: Aspirin and other medications intended for humans should not be given to your dog, except when your vet prescribes it.

- Dog collar: Make sure your puppy's collar is comfortably snug (keeping it "2-fingers" snug is ideal). Always check the fit of the collar to avoid letting it loose and risking your puppy's life.

- Antifreeze: Antifreeze tastes great to dogs, even though it can kill them. At home, secure all antifreeze containers with tight lids and store in a dog-proof area. When up and about, avoid letting your dog step onto puddles.

- Electrical wires: Make sure your plug outlets and electrical wires at home are shielded, and never leave the floors littered with clips, coins, and other such objects.

5. Keep toxic plants out of your puppy's reach.

Animal poison control authorities warn against the following toxic plants:

- All parts of the tomato plant (except ripe fruit)
- Avocado fruit (including pit)
- Corn plant
- Cornstalk plant
- Fig (fiddle leaf)
- Hyacinth bulbs
- Nightshade plants
- Onion
- Peach pits and leaves (wilting)
- Aloe vera
- Baby's breath

- Carnation
- Daffodil
- Geranium
- Hydrangea
- Ivy (branching, English, needlepoint, German, glacier, devil's)
- Hibiscus
- Asparagus fern
- Mistletoe
- Philodendron (whole plant)
- Rhododendron
- Poison ivy
- Poison cloak
- Apricot pit
- Apple seeds
- Bittersweet
- Buckeye
- Calla lily
- Chinese evergreen
- Poinsettia (low level toxicity)
- Cordatum

- Cyclamen
- Dracaena
- English ivy
- Birds of paradise
- Foxglove (digitalis)
- Holly
- Jerusalem cherry
- Lily plants
- Marijuana
- Rubber plant (Indian)
- Narcissus
- Morning glory
- Panda bear plant (Kalanchoe)
- Caladium
- Chinaberry tree
- Easter lily
- Clematis
- Dumb cane and dieffenbachia
- Azalea
- Dragon tree

- Croton
- Elephant ears
- Boxwood
- Oleander
- Hurricane plant
- Plumose fern
- Yew
- Primrose (primula)
- Sago palm
- Wisteria seeds
- Schefflera
- Amaryllis
- Taro vine
- Cycads

Chapter 8

Your Obedience Training Guide

Develop a close bond with your puppy, communicate with him clearly, and allow him to grow well-adjusted and well-behaved with these 5 obedience training tips and tricks.

1. Keep in mind that reward always trumps punishment.

- Reward your puppy for showing the desired behavior. Your dog is most likely to get his obedience training lessons if you make sure to give him rewards for doing something acceptable and desired. See to it that you train your puppy daily and that you reward him accordingly - this teaches him the things you expect him to do. The fact that a dog has not learned means that his owner did not find the time to guide and correct him. Rewarding your puppy for obedience – and with consistency – helps him grow up to become your dream dog someday.

- Set your puppy up for obedience. Let your puppy learn his lesson by choosing to ignore bad behavior and instead setting him up to behave properly and then making a fuss over it.

- Let your puppy know how happy you are with his obedience. Adopt the reward based obedience training technique: Obedience = lovely treats + verbal praise + positive body language.

2. Time is of the essence.

When correcting your puppy out of his disobedience, you need to it immediately as it happens, not long after (when he is likely to forget what he did). Follow up any behavior showing obedience with enthusiastic praise to reinforce said behavior. You can correct your dog's disobedience by interrupting his unacceptable action (different from punishing him) – by tossing a tiny sack of beans or other rattling items, shaking a can filled with coins, spraying water on him, or quickly yanking his leash and then letting it go. Keep in mind that these tactics work best when done with finesse – meaning, your puppy should have no idea that you made the noise or action yourself. The key is to let your puppy think that his disobedience caused the noise or action.

3. Take advantage of your puppy's love for attention.

Your puppy is likely to drop his disobeying behavior if you ignore it. This forces him to switch to a desirable behavior to win back your attention. For example, besides the fact that your puppy loves to carry your smell around, the reason he likes running off with your shoes is that you will look for them later, which results in your giving attention to him. Dogs are like kids, who would rather receive negative attention from you than to be ignored. Allow your puppy to learn his obedience lessons by keeping your personal items (including your shoes) out of his reach.

4. Be on the lookout for chances to misbehave.

- Expect that opportunities to misbehave are always there for your dog. You should take steps to avoid them at all cost. If you do not want your dog to go dashing out the door, make sure to let him learn to follow the "Sit" or "Stay" command first, then have him sit or stay far away while people are coming and going out of the house.

- Make sure you enforce a command before actually giving it to your dog. If you want your dog to come to you, give the command "Come" only after you have attached a long line as his guide to you. Keep in mind that failing to enforce any command only teaches your dog that it is okay not to listen to you and to disobey you.

5. Be clear with your commands.

- Make sure to give any verbal command just once. If you want your puppy to sit, say "Sit" once in a loud voice. If he refuses to follow the command, firmly place him yourself in the sitting position. Never repeat commands (if you need to repeat, it only means your puppy has not learned to "Sit").

- Avoid mixing various commands: If you want your dog to sit, command him to "Sit." If you want him to lie down, say "Down." Never combine the two commands into a "Sit-down" command, this will only confuse your dog. What you can do is to enhance your commands by adding some distractions. If your dog has already learned to "Sit" on command at home, for example, you can try having him follow the same command inside a neighbor's house or out in the park.

Chapter 9

Surviving Your Puppy's First Day at Home

To make your puppy's journey to dream dog-hood even smoother, here are 5 first day survival tips and tricks to guide you:

1. Remember these puppy's first day at home Don'ts.

- Don't forget to give your puppy his new name right away. When changing your puppy's name, make sure to use his new name consistently. This will help him learn it quickly. Help him along by linking his new name first with his old name.

- Don't get mixed signals across. Your puppy might perceive that it's okay to behave badly because you seem to find it entertaining or doing so makes him look cute.

- Don't let your puppy climb up the furniture or bed right away. This is especially important of you still have haven't trained him to recognize you (as well as other members of the family) as the leader in the household.

- Don't issue commands carelessly. You should always be able to issue a command and then enforce it. Your puppy soon learns it is okay to ignore you when you tell him to do something but do not see to it that he follows your command.

- Don't use treats that are too tempting. Such treats include pig hooves or rawhides, over which your dog can fight another animal or even a human because he thinks they will steal his treats away.

- Don't look your dog in the eyes yet. This means, don't place your face anywhere at your dog's eye level and don't attempt kissing him yet. You need to establish yourself as his leader before you position yourself at his eye level, which he might perceive as a threat and give him a reason to bite you.

- Don't keep your puppy away from other people. If you want your puppy to become a socialized and well-adjusted dog someday, then don't even think about letting him stay in the dark. Never put him in dark corners, the garage or basement, or other places that keep him away from family environments.

- Don't teach your puppy to be aggressive. Avoid opportunities for your puppy to learn to challenge you or act aggressive towards you by not playing rough-house, tug of war, and other combative games with him.

2. Make sure all the things he needs are ready for him when he arrives home.

- Crate: You will discover that a crate is an indispensable puppy training tool, especially on your puppy's first day at home. But remember to crate him for no longer than five hours, and make it more puppy-friendly by filling with it with safe toys. For travel, you will find the folding type of crate quite useful, but if your puppy is prone to chewing on crate bars, then an airline crate might be a better option. Choose a crate that will be able to accommodate your pup up to his full adult size.

- Bedding: Opt for puppy bedding that you can easily clean, and make sure that it is made of a thick material that will provide comfort.

- Food and water bowls: Avoid using plastic bowls, as they tend to absorb odors as well as bacteria, which will be harmful to your pet. Make sure to use food bowls and water bowls made with ceramic or stainless-steel material. Do not use of any kind of bowl that has been painted on inside.

- Leash: A twenty-foot dog leash is ideal for training your puppy to follow the "Come" command.

- Dog grooming supplies: Choose the right brush for your puppy's coat. Buy the proper tools for bathing your puppy, as well as cutting his fur and clipping his claws.

- Baby gates: A great confinement alternative to a puppy crate is the use of baby gates. Choose one that your puppy cannot get his paws or head caught in. Make sure to also check if the baby gates you chose are something your dog cannot jump over, knock down, or chew through.

- Pet-specific cleaning products: Choose those that can effectively eliminate dog stains and smells.

- Puppy pen: Puppy pens are also a great alternative to a crate for confining your pup.

- Flea comb: Use a flea comb to check your puppy's coat for fleas. Flea combs also make for good "shedding management" tools.

- Brush: Daily brushing of your puppy's coat may be better for his skin than bathing.

- Bring these when picking up your puppy:
  - ID tag (make sure this is securely attached to your puppy's collar)
  - Leash (made with thick leather/double ply woven and a strong clasp)
  - Buckle collar (made of leather/non-stretched material and with 2-fingers feature)

- Training collar/head collar/head halter/harness (measuring 3-inches more than your dog's neck)
- Crate/carrier (for containing "accidents" while transporting your puppy)

3. Feed your puppy the right food.

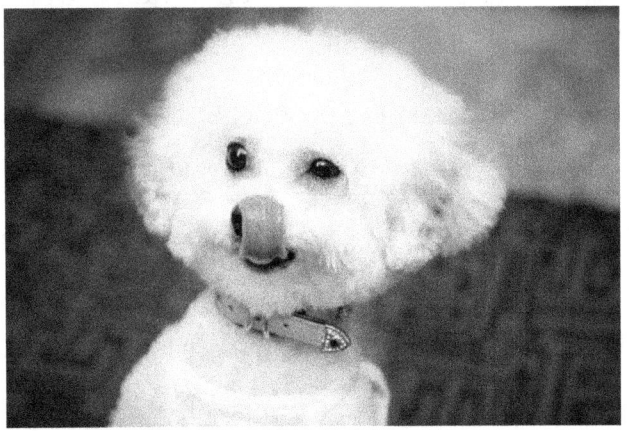

- Make sure to use premium-grade dog food, which goes a long way towards reducing your bills from the vet. Avoid giving table scraps to your dog as this will only encourage him to beg for food, possibly give him indigestion, and lead to weight problems. It also helps to have food items out of his reach.

- You might think you can get away with feeding bargain brands of dog food to your puppy. But these are not necessarily the healthiest food choice for him, possibly costing you more, eventually. Make sure to feed your pup with dog food made with high quality ingredients, and that which contains few allergy-triggering preservatives and byproducts. Remember that dogs are better of eating a consistent diet, so make gradual changes when you do switch dog foods.

- Dry food benefits your dog's teeth by helping keep them cleaner. To ensure that your puppy gets additional nutrients, add baby carrots, green beans, and other fresh veggies to his daily diet. Your puppy would love to have yogurt as well. In case your vet wants to put your puppy on a special diet, make sure to follow through.

- Any digestive issues your puppy might have can be resolved with some plain rice. Meanwhile, the addition of plain yogurt to his food, especially if he is on antibiotics, can help replenish his gut's good bacteria.

- Never allow your puppy to grab food. To discourage this behavior, ask your dog to follow the "Sit" command before feeding him or giving him treats.

- Your puppy could use filter water for its health benefits. Just like humans, he may have some sensitivity to local tap water, and his symptoms may subside after switching him to filtered water.

- Always wash your dog's water bowls and food bowls between feedings. And avoid using plastic ones, which germs love to thrive in.

- Establish a feeding schedule for your puppy; otherwise, you will have to deal with food spoiling and housetraining accidents because of free feeding. In case your puppy is the fussy eater type, take his food bowl after fifteen minutes – don't put it back and just give him food on his next feeding time. You should also keep your puppy away from other animals during feeding to prevent any fights over food.

- Try giving your puppy frozen green beans; they contain few calories, provide nutrients, and are great for chewing on. You may also try adding some apple cider vinegar to your puppy's water bowl daily; it is good for his digestion and even acts as a flea deterrent. It would also be great to supplement your puppy's daily diet with grated parsley, grated carrots, and plain yogurt (low fat).

- You may give biscuits as rewards for your puppy's good behavior; just make sure to give him those made with no food coloring.

- Cook up these recipes your dream dog is sure to love:

- Unstew Dog Meal = Combine raw ground meat (1 pound) with raw liver/gizzards/organ meat (3 ounces), pureed/ground vegetables (2 cups), garlic cloves (2 cloves), ground kelp (1 tablespoon), eggs w/ shells (3 pieces), plain yogurt (1/2 cup), apple cider vinegar (1/2 cup), and parsley (1 palmful); refrigerate or freeze.
- Turkey Loaf = Combine ground turkey meat (3 cups) with old fashioned oats (1 ½ cups), cottage cheese (1/2 cup), eggs (2 pieces), and grated mixed veggies (3/4 cup); press and mold into loaf pan and bake at 350 degrees for 40 minutes; refrigerate/freeze, slice, and serve.
- Cheesy Carrot Chicken Wings = Fill a dog bowl with grated carrots (1/2 cup), cottage cheese (1/2 cup), and raw/cooked chicken wings (5 pieces).

4. Let your dog enjoy his bath time.

- Place a nonslip rubber bathroom mat inside the bath tub. This will allow your puppy to confidently enjoy his bath every time (as opposed to him feeling scared when given a bath because he keeps slipping on the bath tub's slippery surface).
- Avoid using your own shampoo when bathing your puppy. Dog shampoos will do a better job at

cleaning him up, especially since these are made to suit his skin and hair type. Make sure to keep any shampoo away from his eyes.

5. Look after your puppy's dental health.

- Have your vet perform a dental exam on your puppy's mouth as well during each physical exam. Regular dental checkup ensures that the vet is able to get rid of tartar and plaque in your puppy's teeth. Make sure to also have the vet professionally clean your puppy's teeth as needed for his good oral health, which can have a big impact his overall health.

- See to it that your puppy has healthy gums and teeth by regularly brushing his teeth. You can ask your vet for a demonstration on how to brush correctly. Make sure to get doggie dental kits – you should not be using your own toothpaste to brush his teeth.

- If you see any broken teeth in your puppy's mouth, bring him to the vet right away to get the proper medical attention.

- Steps to properly brushing your puppy's teeth:

    1) Secure your puppy to his leash.

    2) Position yourself in such a way that you can easily reach into your puppy's mouth.

3) Squeeze a small amount of dog toothpaste on your clean finger, then let your puppy lick the toothpaste off.

4) Squeeze more toothpaste onto your finger, then massage it gently onto your dog's teeth. You can then use a dog toothbrush as soon as your dog gets used to this step.

5) Reach into your puppy's molars and premolars by gently pulling back his cheeks and lips.

6) Brush your puppy's teeth using circular motions, paying attention to his gum line and back teeth.

Conclusion

Thank you again for purchasing this book!

I hope this book could help you to realize that although training your puppy to become your future dream dog is so much like caring for a human baby – with all the biting and pooping going on – all that hard work is worth all your effort in the end.

The next step is to keep in mind that you are not only caring for a small creature, but an immature animal that needs lots of understanding and training. Prepare to stretch your patience to its limits, and stay realistic and flexible with your training sessions. Allow your puppy to make mistakes along the way, as he is not equipped to automatically learn the training skills you will be teaching him. Lastly, enjoy your puppy's journey and enjoy your time with him!

Finally, if you enjoyed this book, please take the time to share your thoughts and post a review on Amazon. It'd be greatly appreciated!

Thank you and good luck!

www.ingramcontent.com/pod-product-compliance
Lightning Source LLC
Chambersburg PA
CBHW050019230526
45470CB00003B/1047